Think E

CW00420815

Lose Weight From the Top Down

"The proven 3 step formula for lasting weight loss without dieting or going to the gym!"

by

Paul Knight & Mark Benn

Creators of The Slimthinkers Programme

Contents

Chapter 1

A Different Way

"We are what we repeatedly do. Excellence, therefore, is not an act but a habit."

Aristotle

Why do you always end up back at square one?

The thing that is so obvious to us is exactly what the diet and fitness industry doesn't want you to know: if your mind is not on your team then you are doomed to failure and endless yoyo dieting! Fact.

You see, they know you will enter into a diet or fitness regime armed with the greatest of intentions, go so far with your endeavours then quit, or at least revert back to some of your less healthy choices. So you spend time making excuses as to why you failed, get upset to be back where you started or even worse, you live with it for a while then eventually start again! Maybe you found another reason to lose weight or it's the same reason as before. An up and coming event for example, peer pressure, New Year resolutions, getting in to shape for your holiday maybe, the list is endless.

So back to the gym you go, the latest diet book purchased, renewing your subscription to your favourite weight loss group. So more money comes out of your pocket and into theirs! Never-ending cycles that feed the industry, which makes them expand and grow while you are trying to reduce and fit into those jeans again. It's quite ironic that. The industry is built around you failing.

When you concentrate solely on what you put into your body (diets) and what you do with your body (gyms) you are missing one vital component in the equation; your mind. Get the thinking bit right and you will succeed in getting fitter and slimmer. Fact!

But when all you have available to you are diets and gyms, it's no wonder they have the market all wrapped up and you with them. Well it's time to put that problem to bed right here right now! Let us introduce you to a different way. The Slimthinker way! Start at the <u>top</u> and work <u>down</u>! We don't want you to fail.

We wrote this book and created our website for you:

The person who, over the years, has hit the gym and been on countless diets only to find themselves back at square one and feeling like a bit of a failure! Now that's a hell of a lot of people.

Having made that broad statement though, we know from our feedback and research that the typical avatar of the thousands of people we help on a day to day basis, looks something like this:

80% female
Between the ages of 25 and 55
Average weight range 10 – 22 stone
Has low self-esteem and self confidence
Goes on binge dieting periods but has trouble sticking to them
Follows the latest fads and trends with short term results
Feels uncomfortable in a gym environment
Has little time for themselves
Has emotional issues surrounding their weight and food
Wants to lose weight but for the wrong reasons
Isn't ready to change

Are you reading this and grinning to yourself thinking;

"Hey, they are talking about me here! I hate the feeling of being on a diet and sure, I maybe could join the gym, but I really don't want to work with a young trainer who clearly hasn't been overweight in their life so couldn't possibly get what I'm struggling with. A trainer who will put me on a treadmill and watch my bits wobble uncontrollably. What would everyone think? Plus, what with looking after the kids, work and everything else I have to do in a day, all I want to do is chill out when I get the chance at the end of the day, even if it is with a bag of crisps on the sofa watching a soap. And don't even get me started on the subjects of cooking, shopping and food!"

Are you someone who feels under pressure to lose weight? What do we mean by that? Here's a little scenario:

It's December, you know that January is coming up and most of your friends are saying things like "I'm definitely going on a diet after Christmas." You think, well if they are then I better do it too. The TV in January is then full of holiday adverts (making you immediately think of you in a swimsuit) and weight loss products.

Everything you read is geared towards making you feel like you are not doing enough to look and feel better and that you are fat! So you give in and give it a go. But you are not fully committed so you fail and give up. You simply didn't do it for the right reasons and only because everyone else seemed to be doing it. Well rest assured, only a few of those people made it past March too!

Maybe you did decide to lose weight off your own back and went ahead and researched the best way to do it. Big mistake! There is so much stuff out there on the subject (a lot of it completely useless) that you get confused and think, stuff this, and give up before you even start. Maybe you try little bits of everything which ends up being hard work too, as one way of doing something may counter the effects of other advice and teachings.

You may have joined a weight loss group in the past. Not a bad idea you may think as it has its advantages, like being accountable to someone else other than yourself, getting expert advice, meal plans weigh-ins etc. You may have downloaded a calorie tracker or step monitor. All this is great if it works for you. But did it? How far removed from your normal everyday life have these things taken you and what advice did you get to help you make those big changes? What help did you get to tackle the underlying issues that cause you to behave in the way that you do. Habits that have built up over time and got you where you are now?

Our Simple Philosophy...

Change the Way You Think, Move And Eat

It's a simple philosophy but true. If you do the same things all the time, you will get the same results. Fact! So we approach life from a different angle and get different results. Your thoughts control who you are and what you do. Well that's exactly where we start. We work from the head down and not from the backside up like everyone else does.
Once you accept it's your mind that puts your hand in the fridge and it's your mind that puts your trainers on, when you know it's your

mind that decides what you are going to do or not going to do, that it's your mind that will push you on or tell you to give up, you will then realise why you failed in the past and that you can now do something about it. Start at the top, your mind!

Then introduce a different way of moving and eating. That's the way we roll here at Slimthinkers. First change the way you think about yourself and your limiting beliefs, your relationship with food and your life. Then add in simple everyday moving techniques and different eating patterns and Bob's your uncle, easy weight loss that will last. Do you want to fail again?

No. ***So let's start at the top and work down.***

How to use this book to choose a different way

Read the book from cover to cover. Read it again and notice the words in it. Read it out loud and read it in your mind and take action. Do a small thing every day.

To help you focus on this and to help you put it all together, we have also produced the companion e-book for you, which is yours completely free. We will help you start to take control and guide you through the first 2 weeks. Simply take a different approach to your weight loss journey and start from the head down and the rest will follow easily.

FREE 14 DAY STARTER GUIDE COMPANION BOOK

Decide to make small changes today and just sit back and watch the BIG results start to happen!!

Here we guide you step by step. Included in this guide:

- **14 days of mind + behaviour shifts**
- **14 day personal diary**
- **14 day movement plan**
- **14 day snacking guide**

GET YOUR COPY FROM:

www.slimthinkers.com/top-companion-course-book

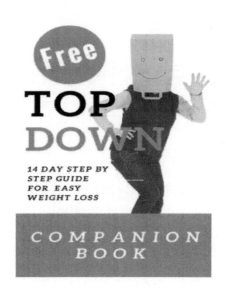

Chapter 2

Tried and Tested

"It does not matter how slowly you go as long as you do not stop."

Confucius

Let's take you back to 2013.

Two very experienced blokes in the weight loss and behavioural change business. One a fitness trainer and weight loss coach, the other an NLP and hypnosis expert. Both with the same objectives in life; *to help people be the best they can be!*

We have known about each other for years but never really got together socially and our paths had never crossed work wise until one day, we found ourselves in the same coffee shop. What was going to be a brief chat turned in to much more. Realising our respective clients would benefit from the other's skills we put our heads together on a number of topics. Our philosophy was born that day.

15 people to take it. It was a physical course, meaning they came to a session once a week for 12 weeks. They would have 1 hour with us and go home with mini tasks to do for the week, along with a hypnosis track to listen to each day.

They all lost weight and there wasn't a diet or a mention of food anywhere. Even we were amazed. It wasn't just weight loss though, but a completely new attitude to life they had all developed. Was it a fluke, we asked? Well we did it again with different groups and with the same results, so no, it wasn't.

Over the next 2 years we listened, reviewed, revamped, re-tested, took things out, put things in, took it online, did it one to one until the present day, 2015. The technology was a bit of an issue but we taught ourselves how to do it so we could deliver our programmes directly in to people's homes. The approach to learning this was the same as the approach to your journey - a little bit at a time. But we learned and put our first website together ourselves. This has allowed us to get our methods out there, and to date, literally thousands of people have successfully taken our courses and changed their habits and behaviours for the better.

From a personal point of view, our own individual knowledge and experience has evolved too, each learning and developing skills and understanding relating to behavioural change and weight loss. An enlightening journey of its own! The most important element being that we are accomplishing our own personal mission;

"To develop a proven method of weight loss that allows people to break the cycle of yo-yo dieting and ends the reliance upon the normal industry standards of losing weight."

Yes there are books, apps, classes, CDs, YouTube channels, clinics and practitioners etc already out there where you can get most of the things you need to turn your life around BUT, where can you find everything you need all in one place and mapped out for you in an easy to follow and easy to do programme that works? One which will save you wasting money and taking up the time you don't have looking for it and then still having to put it all together yourself! There wasn't much out there for you......

Until Now!

Chapter 3

Let's Talk Thinking

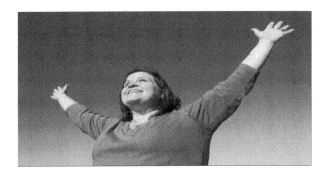

Here is where it all begins. Everything you do in life starts with a thought. Thoughts lead to actions. Thoughts lead to inaction. Thoughts take you forward in life but they can also hold you back!

One of our private clients came to see us. She had been battling weight issues all of her life and she had this problem with crisps, cheese and onion crisps to be precise. Every night whilst watching TV she would munch through 3 or 4 bags! This behaviour is obviously not congruent with a weight loss journey. So what did we do?

We asked what flavour of crisps she *didn't like* and then went about changing the way she thought about the crisps, so that every time she thought about crisps she thought about the ones she *didn't like* and decided to choose a *healthy alternative instead*. This client went on to lose almost 5 stone and got featured in the local press!

Obviously it wasn't just the crisps, there was the issue of why she was eating them, the beliefs she held about herself based on past events and experiences, her current lifestyle, the people she had around her, to name a few. Each one was addressed in small bite-sized chunks, one step at a time. Next, she began to change her patterns of behaviour and beliefs and started forming new ones.

Given the right tools and having the right mindset, it is amazing what we can change in our lives. It is possible to like something once and then something happens and you find you no longer like it. Our minds are just like big computers, following sequences and programmes. We keep repeating these patterns of behaviours every day so in reality, most days of our lives are just replications of previous days.

So how can we change?

All we need to do is create some new patterns or interrupt the existing patterns, forcing us to think in a different way and then repeat the new behaviours for a period of time. However without the desire to change, the desire to wake up and think differently, nothing will ever change. You have to want it to happen.

What did you do when you learned to drive a car? You sat there and took instructions from the driving instructor. At the beginning it was all conscious thought. You really had to think about what you were doing. Each component of driving you had to think of independently because it was new to you. As time passed and you repeated the behaviours, it slowly became embedded into your subconscious mind. The patterns you first had to think about now happen instinctively. You can now work three pedals, a gear stick, steering wheel, indicators, look forward sideways and backwards, judge distance and anticipate others reactions. It took time and focus and a desire to do it. You wanted to drive because it gave you more freedom of movement.

That desire was so strong in you that it drove you forward (pardon the pun). Individual freedom to go where you wanted when you wanted. Driving a car gave you things you didn't have but wanted. Another important thing to consider here is, you didn't stop driving when you passed your test; you carried on repeating the behaviours as part of everyday life without even thinking about it!

When you are on a diet, you are always conscious of it.

Think about it; how many times do you look in the fridge and think, 'no I can't have that I'm on a diet' or, you eat something that is going to put weight on, making you feel guilty because you know you are on a diet! Being on a classic diet is always in your conscious mind. We know that trying to change everything all at the same time simply doesn't work. You can only be successful by making small changes. A Small change but with a BIG impact. We call them TNT moments (Tiny Noticeable Things).

Just a small amount of TNT can make a big bang, right! Being on a classic diet or gym regime is a big change but ultimately not sustainable. It is too far removed from your normal habits and beliefs.

There comes a time when you need to do something different. How do you do that? We use a combination of NLP and Hypnosis. A proven way to get TNT moments happening and sticking.

"Every moment is a fresh beginning."
T.S. Eliot

What Is NLP?

Medicine for your mind.

Have you ever wondered why when you have tried to change a habit or behaviour it usually resurfaces? This is because our conscious willpower usually cannot compete with the power of the subconscious mind.

The subconscious mind is considered to be the source or root of many of our behaviours, emotions, attitudes and motivations. Hypnosis and NLP are powerful tools for accessing the subconscious mind and creating dramatic improvements in our lives.

Neuro Linguistic Programming is a set of specific techniques that deliberately restructure toward positive functioning of the brain's thinking and the body's behaviours. This is done by aligning the conscious and the unconscious mind and body. In other words it's like looking at the patterns and habitual behaviours that we have in life, working out which ones are not congruent with how we want to live and changing them, so they either have a more positive outcome or change the mind body connection. Changing the way you think and feel about all aspects of life.

NLP is a hybrid science that was developed in the late 1960s and early 1970s by computer scientist, Richard Bandler, and linguistic, John Grinder. From the combined perspectives of their respective sciences, they began a study of three therapists, all of whom had excellent results transforming their clients' ways of thinking, feeling and behaving. They modelled family therapist, Virginia Satir, Gestalt therapist, Fritz Perls and hypnotherapist, Milton Erikson, who legitimised hypnotherapy as a healing treatment accepted by the American Medical Association. Bandler and Grinder were looking to discover exactly what transpired in the minds and bodies of patients at the moment change occurred. They asked what specifically caused the change and how this could be replicated more quickly and effectively without years of therapy. These

techniques were modelled and so was born
NLP.

What Is Hypnosis?

Most people have these preconceived ideas
that hypnosis is a state of deep sleep, it is not.
It does involve the induction of a trance like
condition which many people find very, very
relaxing. When within this relaxed state, the
patient is actually in an enhanced state of
awareness, whilst concentrating on the
hypnotherapist's voice. The conscious mind
becomes suppressed allowing access to the
subconscious mind. It is here where real
change can happen. The therapist is able to
suggest ideas, lifestyle adaptations and new
concepts direct to the subconscious, the seeds
of which become firmly planted, enabling real
change to take place at a deep level.

During our sessions you will remain
completely aware of everything that is going
on. In fact, many people experience a hyper
awareness where sounds appear enriched,
thoughts clearer and your ability to imagine
and visualise is greatly enhanced. It is
common for these hypnotic experiences to

create sensations of deep relaxation, fluid warmth or a pleasant tingling sensation or buzz throughout your physical body. Many describe the hypnotic state as a complete and total escape from all physical tension and emotional stress, while remaining completely alert.

By combining the practice of NLP with the delivery of hypnosis, you are more likely to succeed in your desire to make stuff happen in your life instead of letting stuff happen to you. Changing the things you don't want for the things you do want!

Chapter 4

Start Changing Your Mind

What's the problem?

"I want to lose weight but…

"I love chocolate."
"I have no time to focus on me."
"I drink too much."
'I never stick to anything I say I'm going to do."

Do you know someone who doesn't like chocolate? Do you know someone who doesn't drink 2 or 3 glasses of wine a night? Do you know someone who always gets things done? Yes you probably do, so you know it is possible to choose another way of thinking about something and therefore the behaviour that results from that thought process.

If it is humanly possible, it is within your reach.

So what is the issue that always gets in the way? It may be one or a number of things that just gang up on you every time you go down the weight loss path. But why is that issue there? Where did it come from? How do you change it?

To know where we are going we need to know the way, so we start by looking at ourselves and establishing where we are now, that is our starting point.

The Circle of Life. A good place to start.

Grab yourself a pen and a piece of paper and let's begin the change process. Let's start to identify the key areas in your life which need challenging. These areas could be any number of the following:

- Love life
- Relationships
- Partner
- Friends (name them)
- Family (name them)
- Exercise
- Finances
- Work
- Social Life etc

You choose what you want to see on your circle of life.

Draw a circle on your paper. Put a dot in the middle. For each of the areas of your life that you have chosen, draw a straight line from the dot to the outer circle (see the example diagram). Now we need to put some numbers on the lines. Starting with the centre dot as 1, mark 1 to 10 along each line or spoke of the wheel. The number 10 being on the outer circle.

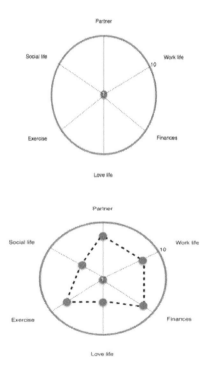

Then score yourself. How do you feel you are doing in your life right now in each area? The number 1 being awful and 10 being amazingly fantastic. Just put a dot on the number you feel is where you are right now.

After you have scored each spoke, connect the dots as shown in diagram. This will highlight the highs and lows of your life right now. Look at the shape it creates, in an ideal world it will be as circular as possible on the outside edge. In other words, your life is as perfect as it could be. That is where you want to get to, a happy circle of life where conflict with others and yourself is looking as good as it gets. It probably won't look like that right now but you have a starting point.

Now choose an area of life from your circle that you want to improve. One of the biggest problems that people have is they try to change everything all at once, so let's take it one step at a time. One emotion at a time. One issue at a time.

Once you have selected the area you wish to improve answer the following questions:

1.   What is the one thing that I could do right now, no matter how small this one thing might be, that will help to change this area? Then do it! NOW.

2.   If it is not humanly possible to do this one right now, set a time and date when you will do it! Then just do it!

As an example, you have picked exercise as an area that is scoring low in your life and you want to improve it. You know you should be doing more and you know you want to do something more, but for some reason you don't. Well number 1 could be...

- Get up now and walk up and down the stairs for 2 minutes - now
- Go for a quick walk - now
- Run around the house with the kids for 5 minutes - now
- Stand up and sit down 20 times then lift something above your head 10 times and repeat this a few times - now

For number 2 (you are on a bus or just going to bed for example) and you can't do it straightaway, decide now to have a quick walk for 5 to 10 minutes and set a reminder now on your phone, When it rings - do it!

Remember, it is what you can do right now, no matter how small, to start making a difference to you. Small changes that will make a big difference repeated over time.

When you have completed each task, revisit your diagram and re-mark the area with your new result and start to watch your circle form. Only tackle one area and one task at a time, remember it's the tiny noticeable things that we do that can make the biggest difference.

TNT MOMENTS

Now you are moving towards becoming happier, identifying your conflicts and then doing small things on a regular basis to reduce the conflict. But what has this got to do with weight loss?

Diets don't work because the root cause or issues in our lives that led to weight gain and the 'want' to lose weight are not tackled. It's your mind that puts your hand in the fridge so, munching on lettuce for a month to lose weight won't work long term. First of all, the chemical reactions and the body's natural instinct to 'store' when the body is restricting its nutrient intake will kick in. The chances are that, after punishing your body and mind for a month with a relentless diet campaign, you will very quickly start to pile the weight back on, because nothing has really changed. You still do or want to do all the things that caused the weight gain in the first place.

It all starts with smiling more, all human beings only want two things in life. The first is to be happy and the second is to avoid conflict.

So what is happiness? Everybody strives for external happiness, - they want to be happy with the world they have created around them - and also internal happiness; happy with oneself, who we are and what we are. It is so important to accept the person that we are and also accept that we can change if the desire to change is strong enough.

Conflict is something else completely, everybody wants to avoid conflict. External conflict with those around us and internal conflict, the battles we have within ourselves.

"Removing conflict from your life creates happiness. When we are in a good place, it enables a stronger focus to enable change to be more effective."

Internal conflict starts with a belief. A belief that you will fail because that's what you have done in the past. A self-belief about yourself that came from somewhere. It was learned from an experience, be that of someone else's making or your own. "You will always be fat, it runs in the family" is a belief planted by someone else. One that stays with you and holds you back from really achieving your weight loss goals. This is then re-enforced in your subconscious mind when you try then fail. "Well maybe Aunty Ethel was right, this is me, get over it."

But you don't want that 'me' and so the conflict begins. The conflict makes you unhappy. Unhappy about yourself, which reaches out into your world until you are unhappy with that too.

The circle of life method starts the process of identifying the issues you have and the ways in which you can start making a few TNT moments to do something about removing the conflicts that are lurking there in your mind.

"Events will trigger emotions that will trigger a behaviour to that event. These behaviours lie in the subconscious mind. The solution is also there, we just need to access it and change it to produce a different outcome."

Overcoming fears, improving your self-beliefs, getting rid of your limiting beliefs, relaxing more, moving more, dealing with stress better, changing your eating patterns, setting goals effectively etc all come in to play. Creating better patterns and habits to live your life by. Starting as of now. As of now you have no problems. Your past was once real and your future doesn't exist yet.

Fractional time in your wardrobe.

When we are asked to explain time, we say look at your wardrobe.

A wardrobe has two doors, imagine one door being your future and the other being your past and that tiny gap in the middle being now, this moment, the second that just happened whilst you are reading this. That second you can't get back and very quickly that second becomes your past! A TNT moment of now that you don't want to waste.

Your 'past' door is heavy and many people carry the past around with them, weight is a feeling. That's your choice, you can live what we call 'backwards' always dwelling on things you know you can't impact or change. They have happened and gone, or you can choose to live now in the moment, this instance. It's your choice, change can only truly happen when you make the decision to change and commit to living towards your future!

Dropping the heavy door of the past and living life in the gap of now. Looking at life this way and understanding that 'now', this moment, is the only reality in your life that we have and we can be sure of. We call it 'fractional time'.

Now is the only reality you have, as of now you have no problems, you are just sitting there reading this. Your past is past and your future hasn't even happened yet! It only takes a second to make a choice. A choice you can make now. Choices are yours to make, no one else's. You make thousands of them every day. What you wear, which way you go to work, how you respond to a comment or situation, Walk or car, chocolate or apple, slouch or sit up straight, do something or put it off...

How do we change our self-beliefs that have built up over time, ones that have created our way of thinking about ourselves and how we behave? Create a goal to move towards this change.

Did you know that in your head right now, you have already started the process? Just by reading this book this far, a new thought process and pathway is beginning to form.

We want you to meet The Choc Monster!

This is a past client of ours. We call him The Choc Monster because that's what he called himself. He had a t-shirt with Choc Monster printed across the chest in big letters. His mates knew him as that and he identified himself with that. He had grown up with this ever expanding waistline and, over time, had made this his identity. It allowed him into the group and to stand out from the crowd. His mates would buy him a pint and a bar of chocolate. He would get them for every birthday and Christmas. He would jokingly say things like, "Oh I don't eat vegetables, I'm The Choc Monster". It was his security blanket but also his excuse. He made all of it believable to himself and others. It was his interpretation of himself and the world around him. To change that behaviour and thinking, he needed to make the belief unbelievable. We come back to The Choc Monster in a minute.

The 3 Veneers

Unless we have a particularly strong public image, we don't have a character list which is available for us to use as a reference point to start building our personality from, so we just make it up! It is best described as the 3 veneers, sometimes referred to as reflections of ourselves.

Inner Self

Who we truly are, is rarely visited and sometimes when we do visit we're not always thrilled with who we find. The inner self harbours all of our most private, deepest thoughts and feelings. We only ever go there when we are completely alone.

Who we think people see and what people actually see!

Our creation - we attach characteristics to this person which we feel best reflects who we think we are or need to be at any particular time. This is best explained when someone comes up to you and says words like "what's up with you today?" and you reply with words like "nothing wrong with me, I'm fine!". Quite obviously in this situation, the character you think you're displaying is being completely misread by the people who actually see you. Life is so much easier if the person you are portraying is the person that people are seeing.

Our own individual interpretation of the world

Ten friends go to a party, they have the same amount to drink, they're all of similar body size, shape and character, they all arrive at the same time and leave at the same time, they all sit on the same table. If this was the case you would think that each individual experience of the party was similar or the same. But what you will find is that a percentage of the people would have a great night whilst others will have an awful night, this is what we find fascinating, it's the same event but vastly different interpretations.

The reason for this is because we all have internal filters for everything that we experience, if we didn't have them our minds would explode with the amount of natural information it would have to filter and sort. So what we do at the unconscious level is ask our minds to search for individual items, experiences or emotions. For example, if you just stop reading this (in a moment) and stare straight ahead, focus on one thing, say the light switch, the information you are processing at that moment is endless; colour, shape, is it on or off, does it have visible screws, which direction are the screw heads facing, how high is it on the wall, is it level, is it clean, dirty or just grubby, what's the approximate distance from the nearest door frame? And that's just for starters. The information that you also have to filter is the wall colouring or is it wallpaper, if it's wallpaper what is the pattern detail and how often is it repeated?

Whatever we choose to look at we only take the detail that we choose to take in the instance that we look at it.

We have all heard of the saying 'if you look for the worst you will find it everywhere' or we say things like 'today is going to be a bad day' and invariably we are correct, because we are asking our minds to search for negative events, emotions and characteristics so we can satisfy the hunt we have sent our minds on. You get what you ask your mind to search for. Take for example, you buy a new car or item of clothing, before you become the proud owner of a green Fiat or a nice slinky red dress you think how wonderfully unique they are. Then suddenly as soon as you take ownership, you see them everywhere. This is because your mind automatically allows these new items through your internal filter system allowing you to see them! This could be the one of the many reasons why people have different interpretations of singular events.

Let's get back to The Choc Monster. The interpretation of his world and his place in it had been formed over time and cemented within his internal filters. His belief is believable because that's what he believes and portrays to others. Others see it and reinforce back to him. Make the belief unbelievable. So what did he do?

His true inner self wanted something different. It wasn't an image or acceptance thing with him but a health and fitness issue. He truly wanted to be fitter and healthier and to stop doing the things that he knew would eventually lead to serious illness. Start believing in such a way that the old behaviour becomes unbelievable. He identified the person who he wanted to be. He saw that person in 3months, 6 months and 12 months' time. He didn't have the t-shirt on. He was more active and he still had his friends and social network. He didn't eat chocolate and he got sportswear for Christmas. He pushed that image in to the front of his mind. It was an image of his creation. A new pattern of behaviour and a different goal. Actually it was a goal, not a new one, as before he just plodded on living life as he saw it and believing what he had created. He didn't have a goal. But now he did and he moved towards it.

So what happened to him? Well last year he went on holiday with his new girlfriend after he had completed a half marathon for charity.

"Value where you are and suddenly where you are will have more value."

In a nutshell...

If it's humanly *possible* it's within your reach. Start changing small things *now*. Focus on *one thing* at a time.

This is the start of a journey using one or two new tools in your tool box. There are many more. The point is, if you do the same things you will get the same result. The mind is the most powerful part of the human makeup. Allowing it to see and do different things allows the new pathways of behaviour to begin.

For downloadable NLP and Hypnotherapy support visit:
http://www.slimthinkers.com/shop/

Chapter 5

Let's Talk Moving

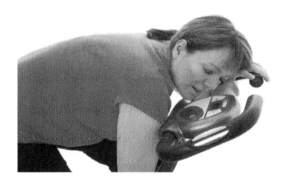

Have you ever entered the words 'how to get fit' into Google and sat there looking at millions of search results all stating that theirs is the best way to get fit and lose weight? The more you search, the more confused you get.

Should I join a class? If so, which class is best? Should I join a gym? Ok, maybe I will go jogging. What trainers shall I get? Do I get a personal trainer? There are hundreds to choose from these days so how do I know they are any good and will I be wasting my money? I know, I will ditch the workout and do Zumba. Actually no, I think I will just stay home and get a workout DVD, they all look so fit and trim on those so it must work, right? I feel a headache coming on!

We have seen trends and fads come and go, some lasting longer than others but the point here is:

"There are no new revolutionary fitness methods out there, just new revolutionary marketing!! It's not called the fitness industry for nothing!"

One thing is for sure, if you are not doing any type of exercise but are still eating cakes, it is a few inches on the butt waiting to happen. What you are going to do from now on is focus on 'mindful movement'. By that we mean everything you do, do it with purpose. The more active you are throughout the day, the more your metabolism is stimulated. The better your metabolism, the better equipped you are to burn calories. Moving with purpose is also linked to the mind. Want to do it, understand why you want to do it and then do it. You want to do it because you are here now reading this.

Exercise is just moving, plain and simple. What do you do when you go to the gym or a fitness class? You move. What do you do when you walk the dog or vacuum the carpet? You move. Remember 5!

Your body is designed to move, to bend and stretch, to lift things, twist, to run and walk, to push and pull. You are doing this all day long or at least at some point in the day. So why do people go to the gym to exercise?

By focusing on what you already do throughout the day and doing it with purpose, you can achieve fantastic results. It's just a matter of increasing your metabolic rate by increasing your activities intensity level. Increase your energy output and stimulate your body's natural fat burning furnace. <u>Remember 5.</u>

The point here is, move with purpose, get you heart beating a little faster and get out of breath as many times as you can throughout the day. But how do you do it, what do you do, how much time will it take and when should you do it? With our expert guidance, you can be moving purposefully and losing weight without having to add an exercise class in to the mix. Bargain.

Time and Exercise

We keep mentioning the number 5. It's an important number to say, think about, remember, look at and notice. It will become part of your subconscious mind and part of the new path you are creating. Five. Time is one of the most used excuses for NOT doing any form of exercise. Before we get to that one though, let's mention some of the others;

"I can't afford it."

Well, if you think of exercise as going to a gym or class then there's a considerable cost and commitment involved. Being mindful will cost you nothing! Plus there are no travel costs or expensive gym wear or equipment to buy. So that one just went out the window! Remember 5!

"I'll do it when."

If you're waiting for the right time to start doing a bit of exercise you will be waiting a long time. But, again it boils down to what you think exercise is. Getting your heart rate up and overloading and stretching your muscles for 5 minutes at a time doesn't need that much to change in your life, so why wait? Remember 5!

"I'm too tired."

The more time you can include into your day for exercise (movement), the less tired you will feel! Energy levels will be increased and maintained throughout the day, sleep patterns will improve and that sluggish 'can't be bothered' attitude will take a back seat. Remember 5!

"I'm too fat."

No you're not, sorry you can't use that one either. Yes it may be harder to start because you are carrying extra bits around with you but any exercise can be modified to help you get moving. **Remember 5**!

There are more excuses where these came from, but at the same time, there are more answers too. That applies to anything in life, not just exercise.

5

THE 5 MINUTE PRINCIPLE

Probably the biggest excuse of all is this one; "I simply do not have the time". Given modern living and the hectic lifestyles that most people lead these days, this is a sticky one. So we want to take some time and work with you on this one for a while.

There are 24 hours in a day, no arguing with that fact! Let's say the average time spent in bed sleeping is 8 hours. That leaves you 16 hours in a day to move. Now, if you go along the lines of going off somewhere to do a fitness session, it means that you have 16 opportunities in your busy day to fit it in. Is that feasible? For some the answer is yes, for most it's no. Ok so let's break it down a bit further.

Let's say that your exercise regime involved just 30-minute sessions. You just doubled your chances of fitting something in to a more manageable 32. That's 32 opportunities to do a 30-minute exercise routine in your busy day. It's looking a little better now isn't it? Can you do that? The answer is still probably "maybe not guys, sorry". Let's keep going and reduce your activity to 15-minute slots.

Again you have doubled your chances of moving your ass to a massive 64! Can you spare just 15 minutes out of the 64 you have just made available to you? The answers are getting more like yes now rather than no! Here's where it gets even harder to say, "No I don't have the time".

Just imagine if you could do your exercise sessions in 5-minute spurts (remember you have been remembering 5!). That means there's now a whopping 192 opportunities in a day to do something about how you look and feel! Really, we hear you say. How do I do that? Glad you asked.

"192 chances to do 6 x 5 minutes bursts of movement!"

But what is fitness anyway?

Well let's start by saying what it is not.

It's not a once every now and again thing you do every January 1st or before you go on holiday. It's not just something you do to look good, that's an added benefit of being fit and active. We are not talking here about fitness for running a marathon, but simple fitness for everyday life and health that will help maintain weight loss and positive mindsets. *Put simply, being fit means being able to do the things that need to be done in your life without feeling knackered 2 minutes in to doing it!*

Fitness is relative to the individual. Having enough puff in your lunges, strength and flexibility in your body to be able to do whatever you want to do. As a result you will feel better, cope better, sleep better and weight and shape will begin to change. Know that by moving consistently over time your body will be making positive changes and results will come.

Fitness starts with a decision. A decision to do something about it for a reason. Let's say as an example... to be able to kick a ball around the garden with your kids for 10 minutes a day. Then make a plan. Keep it real and keep it simple. This plan does not involve watching the football on the TV to pick up kicking and dribbling techniques. Start by actually doing it for 2 minutes and increase it by 2 minutes every day until your dazzling Beckham-like skills last for the 10 minutes and it's the kids that give up first because they can't get the ball off you!

Starting any exercise and fitness plan to lose weight can be a very real motivator, but picking something that is fun and enjoyable is maybe better, as shape and weight loss are a by-product of moving more and eating better.

So where do we start?

Chapter 6

Mindful Movement

"Nothing happens until something moves."
Albert Einstein

What we know so far in a nutshell:

Exercise is just moving. There are no excuses. You have 192 opportunities in a day to move and start burning the fat off.

Let's take a moment here to consider whom this book is written for. The people out there who feel uncomfortable in a gym environment, don't actually like exercise, or who don't have the time to go there on a regular basis. Normal everyday people, living normal everyday life and who want to lose some weight and feel better about themselves. It will however benefit those of you who do train on a regular or semi-regular basis and the principles can be incorporated in to your days too.

To get the principle of 5-minute workouts in to your head a little better, we have taken extracts from the NHS and UK Government websites on the subject of health and fitness.

Here's what they say:

- Adults should aim to be active daily. Over a week, activity should add up to at least 150 minutes (2½ hours) of moderate intensity activity in bouts of 10 minutes or more – one way to approach this is to do 30 minutes on at least 5 days a week.

- All adults should minimise the amount of time spent being sedentary (sitting) for extended periods. Minimising sedentary behaviour may include:

  - reducing time spent watching TV, using the computer or playing video games, taking regular breaks at work.

  - breaking up sedentary time such as swapping a long bus or car journey for walking part of the way.

What are the benefits of being active daily?

Reduces risk of a range of diseases, eg coronary heart disease, stroke, type 2 diabetes.

Helps maintain a healthy weight.

Helps maintain ability to perform everyday tasks with ease.

Improves self-esteem.

Reduces symptoms of depression and anxiety.

The end.

This means that, if you were active in 5-minute bursts 6 times in the day (remember that's only 6 out 192), you will have done your 30-minutes exercise session before you go to bed! Bargain! You can do that can't you? The question is how?

Mindful movement - turn everyday life into a gym workout!

It's about moving with purpose whenever and wherever you get the chance. No one needs to know you are doing it. Just move with purpose. Put you mind to the task for just five minutes, focus on the activity or situation you find yourself in and, while you are being mindful of your body, move with purpose!

What changes, no matter how small, could you make to your day, your actions, your thoughts or your environment?

Mindful movement can be broken in to 2 sections - one where you just do it, whatever it is, and the other is planned, making the time.

The Purposeful 5

As you read this, how are you sitting? Slouching, no doubt. Correct your posture now then! Change the way you sit. Consciously draw you belly button in to your spine as you breathe out and tighten your abs. Sit up straight! You will be surprised how much that will begin to create a difference and become a habit. It may seem a little crazy to suggest that just sitting differently works, but try this as one of your 5-minute mindful movements (even though you are not moving) slots:

Sit on the floor with your back against a wall. Have your backside, middle and upper back, shoulders and head, in its natural position, gently pressed against the wall as you sit up straight for a few minutes. Relax your shoulders and gently draw your belly button in to your spine every time you breathe out. You will soon begin to feel the muscles in your body begin to work because you are finally thinking about using them properly!

So a subtle change in sitting and breathing is a start. We can all manage that right? You could do it as you sit watching the TV for instance or in a lunch break. You are sitting everyday so just do it with purpose and be mindful of how you do it. It is a great little exercise that no one knows you are doing and will go a long way to helping you improve your posture. If your posture improves then so does your confidence.

Let's take another thing you do every day – walking. It's as simple as putting one foot in front of the other. You have been doing it since you were a toddler. Walk as if you are late 3 times a day for 5 minutes at a time. Walk as if you are late. Get your heart rate up and be slightly out of breath. Walk faster than you do normally. Do it mindfully for 5 minutes. Walk purposefully 3 times a day. Put one foot in front of the other as quickly as you can. Focus on this wherever you find yourself. Focus for 5 minutes and keep it there for 5 minutes. All you have to do is walk with purpose for 5 minutes and repeat that pattern 3 times a day. You do it anyway. You will get closer to your goal with every step you take. Fact! You walk anyway so make it work for you.

So sit up straight and walk like you're late!

That's just 2 TNT moments that you can choose to have for yourself right now. You won't get them back once they are gone!

Becoming more mindful and purposeful is the key to movement (exercise) and allows you the opportunity to fit it in to your normal everyday life. It is not a change to your routine that you will eventually stop because it is so far removed from normal living, especially if you are not enjoying it and doing it under duress. It's just a focused and simple addition and a mind change. It's just forming a simple habit. Here's an example of just one way you can get your metabolism firing and working for you even before you have go to work in the morning:

You get up, have a stretch and a yawn, probably go for a wee first then head for the kitchen. You fill the kettle up and flick it on. You then pop a tea bag in a cup and pop some porridge into the microwave. As the kettle boils you do this; circle your arms a few times, swing your arms across your chest and fling them out wide to the sides a few times. You then do a few leg swings forward and back while you hold on the kitchen counter. Now you feel a bit more awake.

You then do 30 seconds of standing pushups on the kitchen counter followed by 30 seconds of squats still holding onto the kitchen counter for support (or not if you can).

You pick up the milk (with the top still on of course) and holding it in both hands, lift it up and down above your head for 30 seconds. Then you repeat the whole thing again once or twice. We call this 'the kettle wait'.

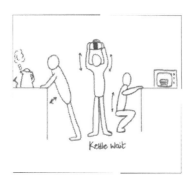

Kettle Wait

You have your drink and porridge and head to the bathroom to wash. As you clean your teeth you look at yourself in the bathroom cabinet mirror. As you stand there with your feet shoulder width apart and your knees slightly bent, you do a side bend so you can't see yourself anymore. Return to the stand, see yourself and then bend the other way. We call these the 'peekaboo'.

You go get dressed and head for the car. As you drive, you sit up straight and gently pull you belly button in towards your spine for as much of the journey as you can, at least 5 minutes anyway. We call them 'car tummy tucks'.

What did you just do?

You stimulated your metabolism and made it go higher. You ate breakfast and stimulated your metabolism even more. You worked your back, shoulders, chest, arms, legs and tummy muscles. You did 2 out of the 6 little workouts you are going to fit into your day even before you got to work! You did the kettle wait, peekaboos and the car tummy tucks. You were mindful of what you were doing and what you wanted to achieve as you did them with purpose. You made a conscious decision that will form an unconscious behaviour that you will repeat on a regular basis. You made a start. A start to a positive day ahead and a start to getting where you want to be!

Is it that simple, we hear you say? Well yes it is! Purposeful, mindful and focused movement throughout the day every day will be conscious behaviour for a while, then you won't even notice you are doing it. And the best part is, for someone who has a fear, an aversion or a complete lack of interest in exercise, you will probably burn more calories and get fitter than the average Joe that attends the gym 3 times a week!

The Planned 5

Now we don't know you or your circumstances or abilities. We will include 3 exercises in this section and how to do them and then how to fit them in to your day. You can get more exercise to suit you and your needs everywhere, so we will leave that up to you. We just want you to get the habit.

Make the time or use the time. In other words, you may find yourself with a bit of time on your hands at some point in the day. So why not use it? Get 5, 10 or 15 minutes of quality movement in. The other scenario would be planning your exercise time.

Be flexible in your thinking. For example, sometimes it's easier to group your favourite mini sessions together for say a 15 minute workout at lunch with a 10 minute session before work and say 5 minute abs at night. Other days may not suit this routine so mix it up! As long as your sessions total 30 minutes from the time you get up to the time you go to bed it's entirely up to you when you fit it in.

Some days may present a free morning where you could actually do 5 mini workouts straight through. Just look at your day(s) ahead and figure it out in advance. Put reminders on the wall, fridge, your phone or computer. Anything that will jog your memory that it's time for five! Alternatively, keep your workouts to hand and whip one out when you have a free five! Go it alone or better still get your friends and colleagues to join in with you. Make it fun.

Every 5 means 5 minutes of you time. 5 minutes of taking a step forward and planting a seed in your subconscious mind. A habit that is moving you in the direction you want to go. 5 minutes of you time. Making you fitter, stronger and slimmer. A TNT moment (or 5!). A conscious moment of movement that has itself come from a subconscious thought. A habit. A change you are making right now. Now is all that matters.

So, let's give you a hand...

A simple 5 minute workout you can do anywhere with no equipment. First of all we will show you a few simple exercises and then how to put them together.

Press Ups

Keep the body strong and straight throughout the move. Ensure a straight line from the shoulders down through the hips to the feet. Lower the whole body towards the floor, chest to an imaginary line drawn between the hands until the arms are at a 90 degree angle. Breathe out on the way up.

Remember the easier version is to do it on your knees (2) or against a table (1).

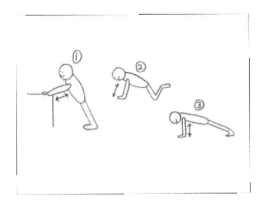

Squats

Feet shoulder width apart. Squat to a 90 degree angle at the knees keeping your back flat, knees behind your toes, heels on the floor and shoulders in line with your feet. Push up through your thighs to stand. As you do this breathe out, pull your belly button in to your spine and squeeze your thighs and buttocks at the top on the move.

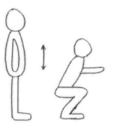

Sit Ups

Lying on your back with knees bent and feet on the floor, bring both knees towards your belly button and your chest towards your knees. As you do this breathe out and pull your belly button in towards your spine. Return your feet and shoulders to the floor.

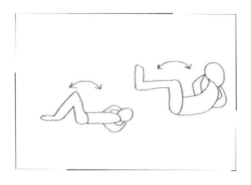

Now in addition to these 3 simple exercises we want you to add in a stair walk. All that means is walking up and down your stairs. If you don't have any at your place then find a step and just step up and down on that. If you can't find one then do something 'aerobic' like dance to your favourite music, pretend you are in the ring with Ali and shadow box. Anything that will help to get you out of breath and a bit of a sweat on!

Now let's put it together in 5 minutes.

You are going to do a circuit training session. This means that, after a little bit of a warm up, you will do 30 seconds of each exercise one after another for a total of 5 minutes. Try not to take a rest between each one but instead move straight into the next 30 second slot. In that 30 seconds put your 100% in to it, whatever that means to you. Do as many of each exercise as you can within the time. Each day you do it, try and beat the amount you did the last time. Simple. Focus on the correct technique and breathing and just do it. Have fun doing it and know that it's a TNT!

"Ensure you warm up and cool down. If you are new to exercise please take it easy to start with and build. Consult a doctor if you need to before commencing."

Warm up

This is simply getting your body ready. Circle your arms, take your arms across your chest then fling them out to the sides. Hold on to something and gently swing a leg forward and backwards through a comfortable range of movement. Stand for a few seconds and alternate flicking your heels up towards your backside. That's all.

Now just follow this......

1. 30 secs press ups
2. 30 secs squats

3.   30 secs sit ups
4.   30 secs aerobic (the stair run or
     something to get you puffing)
5.   30 secs press up
6.   30 secs sit ups
7.   30 secs aerobic
8.   30 secs press up
9.   30 secs squats
10. 30 secs aerobic

Now have a little stretch and drink some water
and you are done.

By following this simple strategy of mindfully
moving with purpose in your everyday life and
combining it with a few planned 5 minute
sessions with yourself, you will be amazed at
how quickly your mind and body begin to
work together. As we have mentioned
previously, peoplc who do this consistently
and make it a habit have a better outcome
than those attending a gym 3 times a week.
The reason is this:

Constant movement keeps the mind and body
focused. Going to the gym will have its
benefits true, no doubting that. But how many
times do those people lapse? In other words,

how long do they keep it going? It's back to the stop start scenario. Plus, when folks are 'training', they get in the mindset of "ah well I can have this huge chunk of chocolate or junk food because I'm going to the gym tomorrow and will burn it off".

So small habitual moments of movement work. You do not have to go anywhere to do them, spend any money or run the risk of stopping. It hasn't taken you away from your normal everyday life as you have incorporated it in to it.

Exercise to lose weight is just movement and it only takes 5 minutes of focus!

Chapter 7

Let's Talk Eating

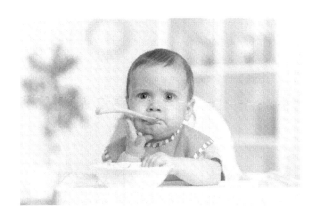

Diets fail for a number of reasons.

The main reason we have found in our years of teaching is this: if you want it and you can't have it you want it more. So by default, this is telling us we are punishing ourselves and it becomes a chore and causes internal conflict. So we end up going back to our usual behaviours. We look at food in a different way. Be aware, this is not a diet book, we don't get people hung up on dieting. We just want you to change your thinking.

Have you noticed how many diet and cook books there are out there? The trouble is, the diet book you just bought has just told you that the food you just learned to cook in your new cookbook is bad for you! Ah well.

You are a chemistry set and what you put in to your body determines how your body functions. This is not going to be a chemistry or biology lesson; we just want you to understand this concept. What you put in has an effect on what happens. What needs to happen is simple; you need to burn off calories and fat by making your body behave in that way. To make it work for you all day and every day, just feed it the chemicals it needs to get the job done. Good chemicals from good food. Food that looks like food and doesn't come from a lab.

"Don't dig your grave with your own knife and fork."
English Proverb

Some foods will speed up your metabolism and others will slow it down. Some foods will help keep your cravings at bay, others will keep you feeling fuller for longer. The food industry is a minefield. You need a PHD to read a food label. The weight loss industry is even worse. Just because it says low calorie, and the picture on the label looks inviting, doesn't mean it will help you lose weight. Let's keep it really simple.

First of all it's understanding why you do things and how to change them. Why do you sit at home and snack on the things you know for sure are not good for you? Laziness, boredom, reward, lack of motivation? You do it because that's what you do, it's your current pattern of behaviour.

Why do you blame lack of time in preparing the food you take on board? That's the reason you always opt for the convenience food. You do have the time if you manage your time better. This relates to breakfast too, you don't have it because you think you don't have the time. A 5 minute breakfast is easy.

The way you eat is a major factor in losing weight too, not just simply what you eat. You may be someone who eats even when you are full. You carry on eating because you don't recognise the full signals your brain sends to your stomach and vice versa. You eat 'til your plate is empty because of the patterns of behaviour that have been instilled into your subconscious over the years since you were a child.

You eat because your brain sometimes doesn't differentiate between being hungry or being thirsty. Thirst and hunger are closely related. Being hydrated therefore is a must for this and many other reasons.

A shopping trip is where it all begins. If you don't put it in the basket to take home it won't be in the cupboard when you get the call to run to it.

Then it comes back to the chemistry set!

Let's kick this off with eating habits.

You have no doubt had this done to you when you were a kid and probably done it yourself to your kids too. When a baby or a toddler is full or doesn't like the food it is being offered, it will say no. Turning the head away from the food, closing its mouth and turning up its nose. It goes purely on what it wants, what it needs and what it likes. It doesn't go by a clock, it doesn't know when it's lunchtime. Their body tells them. And when they eat they are focused on the process of eating.

Now move on a bit. The parent then tries to force the child to eat 'til the plate is empty. "Just one more mouthful, here it comes" and the parent makes 'choo choo' noises. "Eat this and you can have extra playtime before bed", so reward is associated with clearance of the plate. "If you don't finish your dinner you can't have pudding", there's punishment thrown in to the mix, which is associated with eating more than you need.

So from an early age you have been fighting an upward battle with what you need, what you eat and the emotional factors of reward and punishment associated with food clearance.

Successful weight loss starts here.

Chapter 8

How to Eat to Lose Weight

Let's stick with eating like a baby and making it a mindful experience. Begin to notice the full signs. As we mentioned before, a baby will tell you when it is full. Let your *inner baby* do the same for you.

It takes a while for the food in your stomach to register in your brain and then your brain to tell your stomach that it is full. If you are eating on the go, in a rush, while watching TV and not really concentrating on the act of eating, your mouth and mind are not in sync. Slow the process of eating down. Digestion actually starts in the mouth where food is broken down by mixing with the enzymes in saliva, making it easier for the stomach to handle.

Make time for eating. Set a time aside and do just that, eat. A park bench, the dinner table, wherever. Put your knife and fork down between mouthfuls and don't load them up with the next mouthful ready to go in. Have water before you eat and importantly, take regular sips after every other mouthful of food. Water is key in so many ways. It is the secret weapon in weight loss.

Have you ever noticed how you start moving food around on your plate as you start to feel full? You might take a big breath, shuffle in your seat or adjust your clothing. These are all signals you are getting to the limit and you should think about the next forkful. Do you actually need it? Is the process of nutrition complete for that sitting? Begin to notice the full signs in yourself and others.

You can make one choice easily *now,* or a number of much harder choices later. By this we mean, choose not to put crap in your shopping basket once, and the need to make choices at home at night in front of the TV, won't have to be made. You know what it's like when you say "I will only have 3 pieces of chocolate instead of half the bar tonight". After the 3 pieces, do you stop? The next evening the same conflict in your mind arises and the battle continues. If it is not in the cupboard you don't have those choices to make. At the point of purchase you have a stronger mindset than relaxing at home after 8pm, providing you are not shopping while you are hungry that is!

The best ready meal you can ever choose to eat is the ready meal you got ready yourself! Yes, time can be an issue sometimes but time is yours. You make the time, you use the time. Prepare to succeed. Remember the 5 minute rule for moving? Well it doesn't stop there. It applies to all aspects of your life. It takes 6-7 minutes to hard boil an egg. While you are doing that, chop up some fruit and veg and stick it in to a container for the next day along with a piece of chicken you cooked last night for example. Make the healthier choice now so you don't have to settle for something that comes through your car window the next day because you take the "can't be bothered" route. Better choices, better outcomes. Small decisions and behaviours that become the norm when repeated over time.

> *"The best ready meal you can ever choose to eat is the ready meal you got ready yourself."*

Some of our clients go down the route of smoothies and soups. Once prepared and perhaps frozen, these are another source of good homemade ready meals. The nutritional values of the products being 'smoothed or souped' may be slightly less than if it is eaten raw, but they are a definite improvement on the ready meals you will find out in the world of supermarkets, petrol stations and local convenience stores when you just grab and go. Create the behaviour and repeat.

Breakfast, yes or no?

There are countless research projects into the pros and cons of eating breakfast and its effect on your weight loss journey which includes your general health and wellbeing. Having worked in this industry for many years, we have come to understand that eating something nutritious in the first hour of getting up from a hopefully restful sleep is a must. This is known to all as breakfast.

Having breakfast will help provide the energy, vitamins and nutrients you need to start the day, help stop the desire to snack on something sugary mid-morning and helps you make better food choices during the rest of the day. It sets the tone for the rest of the day, it gives you a head start and a positive step forward. A small habit that is making a huge difference.

"I don't have time for breakfast and what do I need to eat anyway??"

Here's what we do and more importantly what our clients do. Notice the nutrients and protein included into these two simple options...

Quick up and out – put kettle on, put porridge into the microwave, get frozen blueberries out of the freezer and run a handful under the hot tap. Make a green tea, take porridge out and add the blueberries, a sprinkle of cinnamon and a spoon of honey. Eat. Time 10-15 mins all in, tops. Head out the door with your ready meal and a bottle of water.

More time option – Scramble some eggs and add in some salmon shavings. Add a slice of toast if you wish. Have a yogurt with chopped up fruit and a few nuts. A drink of your choice. Head out with your water and ready meal.

If you are not already including breakfast in your day, creating the habit is the same as always; baby steps one at a time until you have it cornered. Do it for a couple of mornings to start with if you wish and add more days to the habit as you go. Think about it, plan it if needed or just do it. Even if it is as simple as eating a piece of fruit with your tea or coffee before you rush out the door. The important part is to first create the physical routine. As your mind and body begin to sync and the routine becomes the norm, you will automatically begin to think more about the content of the habit.

The Dreaded Night Time Snacking!

THE most common eating pattern which has the most detrimental effect on weight loss is the dreaded night time snacking. We get so much feedback in this one subject that we have created and delivered a mini course on it!

"I'm so good and focused through the day, watch what I eat and what I do, then screw it all up after 8.00pm when I get the munchies and start nibbling and the wine comes out." A quote from a client which has been repeated by many in different ways.

Remember the client who ate 4 bags of crisps every night and went on to lose 5 stone? We helped her choose not to. Not only changing her thoughts on the crisps, but her pattern of behaviour around that time of night and before. Here's what she did...

She closed the kitchen at a certain time every evening. This meant making and putting a 'closed' sign on the kitchen door. She spent time on that sign, putting all the wants and desires in to it as she drew it and coloured it in. The person she wanted to be wrote it, not the person she was trying to get away from. The sign interrupted her thoughts and normal patterns, changing her behaviour if she went near it. When you have finished your evening meal, make a conscious effort to tidy the kitchen, put everything away where it should be. Then, before retiring to the lounge, TURN OFF THE LIGHTS and CLOSE THE KITCHEN DOOR and say out loud "THE KITCHEN IS NOW CLOSED".

She stuck a picture of a dress she wanted to wear but couldn't fit into on the fridge door. She put a time, place and date on the fridge when she would be wearing it. After her evening meal she had a cup of green tea and then cleaned her teeth. It worked. Green tea helps take the cravings for sweet things away. Cleaning your teeth signals to the brain that eating has stopped and it's time for bed. All of these things she added in over time, small changes, TNT moments that made the big difference.

Before she even got to this stage, we encouraged her to plan her snacking. Her 'addiction' to the crisps and the emotions around the act were too strong to just snap out of. We asked her to put the crisps into a bowl and eat them from there. She could see them and noticed them. She made a conscious decision to eat slower and not so many, even sharing them. A planned act that was better than the one she was previously doing. She began to sip on water too as the evening approached. Filling her up and hydrating her. A small 500ml bottle of water on the arm of her chair.

It's the tiny things you change that make the big impact 'TNT'.

So in a nutshell...

Start the day right, take <u>your</u> ready meal with you, cook at night then choose not to snack after dinner. Drink 6 bottles of 500ml water a day and sip on it through meals too. Shop with all this in mind and make the decisions when you are feeling strong! A different eating pattern. A better way of eating. A different way of eating that will produce the desired result, weight loss. Use the time you have. Remember the 5 minute rule and apply it to all aspects of your life.

There are 2 ways of losing weight;

Eat less calories and move more to use the calories you are eating or to increase your metabolism.

There are 2 ways to increase your metabolism;

Internal burn and external burn. Internal being the food you eat and external being the movement you make during the day.

Both ways focus on a balance of in and out, but counting calories is boring, restrictive, punishing to the mind and ultimately leads to failure in many cases.

With our clients we focus on what will speed you up and what will slow you down. Oats speed you up, wheat slows you down. Sitting slows you down, moving speeds you up.

Here's a simple equation to put that into your mind, see it in your mind, notice it and let it sink in.

The 3 part equation

Move + Eat + Think = Internal and external met burn = Weight loss

Chapter 9

What To Eat To Lose Weight

If the food you have in the cupboard has a shelf life of months and months, then it's probably not food. If the food in your cupboard has ingredients in it that you can't pronounce with a few numbers and letters after them, it's probably not food. If you're going to eat animals, eat the ones that have eaten well themselves. This applies to the things like eggs too. Just a few little thoughts on food there you might want to take note of and notice.

Everyone is different with a different body make up. The best 'diet' for you is the one you come up with yourself. What works for you. What are your individual tastes and hates? We don't live with you. We don't know you. Unless you have been living on Mars this past few years, you will already have a good idea of what is good for you and what is bad. Yes the so-called experts do change the goal posts every now and again, having done a government or food industry leader funded research project, but the basics stay the same.

When we take a client on a supermarket shopping trip, we spend a lot of time on the fresh food aisles picking colours, tastes and textures. Things that go well together, things that are easy to prepare and quick to cook. Things that are grown from the earth or things that have eaten from the earth. Things that have been pulled from the sea. We then head for the frozen section and look for the same kind of things that have been frozen close to the point of picking or catching. We go looking for the bottles of water they will need and the spices and herbs etc. they can add to their meals. Food types that will be easy to prepare and cook. Food that will help their metabolism fire up. Remember 6 bottles of 500ml is a rule to follow for water.

Yes they are allowed the processed easy to cook or microwave foods that are there, but they fill only the tiniest space in the trolley. You know, the smaller space sectioned off at the front of the trolley. They know it's not food and it's not good for them, but if they want it they have it. It's their choice, as it is yours too. Apply the 80/20 rule. 80% of your choices being the healthiest and 20% from the 'oh sod it' aisles!

Remember this is not a diet. Eat what you want, just know why you are eating it and what it's doing for you (or to you!).

Homework!

As you will probably have guessed by this point in the book, we are not about dieting and conventional thinking with regard to weight loss. We are not going to start now by telling you what to eat, instead we will just point out a few things you need to notice. Notice and take note of. Notice and be mindful of the tricks and traps you may fall into. Traps laid by others that want to make money, regardless of whether it is good or bad for you.

Proteins, carbs, vitamins, fats and minerals, all play a part in our health and function. The elements of the chemistry set we mentioned before, all are to be included in our daily intake of food. Yes even fats. It's all about balance.

A quick word about bread.

We have, as a species, eaten bread as a staple part of our diet for years. Nowadays, commercial growing and baking of mass quantities for the modern supermarket shelves have replaced much of the natural processes - instead being replaced with the additives. This is one of the major factors in the now common ailments of bloating and IBS etc. Gluten has become the enemy for thousands and thousands of people worldwide. We have yet to come across anyone who has not felt better when they have cut down on or cut out completely, popular branded sliced bread. If you do want it, buy freshly baked or pitta, ciabatta etc. Remember, wheat slows you down, it's like putting glue in your engine.

Back to the homework. To start the process off, we want you to take note of what is in your food stores now. Cupboards, freezer and fridge. The secret hiding places too! Many people buy the same stuff all the time, replacing that same food stuff when it runs out. Take a moment over the next few days to read the labels. Google 'how to read a food label' for example and see exactly what's in it. Remember, just because it says low calorie doesn't mean it's helping you lose weight. Just like the 'closed' sign on the kitchen door, this action helps break the thought and habit process of just throwing what you normally do in the trolley next time you go shopping. If you are looking to lose weight why would you continue to continually eat the same things in the same quantities?

Shop backwards. Start in a different place in the store and chose a different route around it. Likewise, take some time to move things around in the kitchen. Put things where they are not normally kept. Disrupt the pattern! Your subconscious knows where things are, its way around the store and where your usual stuff lives. Make it a conscious act to shake things up a bit to create new habits and behaviours.

The next thing is to start jotting down what you eat and how it makes you feel.

Remember the circle of life? Food is an area of your life that may need your attention. There's no need to make this too complicated though. Just start to be aware of what's going on in your life in a visual way. Be honest and write it down. Give yourself a starting point and something to look back on. Where do you score, what can you do right now. What small step can you make to improve what you are eating? A small swap perhaps. Water instead of juice or fizzy drinks perhaps. Keep it simple and repeat it over and over again. Then make another choice and take another additional step. An ongoing process of change instead of a sudden and complete change, one that feels like a punishment and not something that is good for you.

Begin to notice what you are currently doing, your eating habits and the food that is regularly being put in to our body. Don't follow a diet but instead, begin to understand what the various types of food groups do for your body, the chemistry set. For example protein.

Proteins are the main building blocks of the body. They're used to make muscles, tendons, organs and skin. Proteins are also used to make enzymes, hormones, neurotransmitters and various tiny molecules that serve important bodily functions. Without protein, life as we know it would not be possible.

Proteins are made out of smaller molecules called amino acids. Some of these amino acids can be produced by the body, while we must get others from the food we eat. The ones we cannot produce and must get from our foods are called the "essential" amino acids.

Protein is incredibly important when it comes to losing weight.

As we know, in order to lose weight, we need to take in fewer calories than we burn. Eating protein can help with that, by boosting your metabolic rate (calories out) and reducing your appetite (calories in). This is well supported by science. But probably the most important contribution of protein to weight loss, is its ability to reduce appetite and cause a drop in calorie intake. Protein is much more satiating than both fat and carbs.

In other words, by adding more protein to your daily food intake, you will feel fuller for longer. The amount of energy required to digest the protein is greater too so you are using more calories (higher metabolism and the thermic effect of food). Protein helps in muscle building and therefore provides a better ratio of muscle to fat in your body composition. Muscle burns more calories even at rest. And that's not all. Eating more protein has been shown to reduce cravings and desire for late-night snacking. Just eating a high-protein breakfast may have a powerful effect. Take an interest in your food and find out more yourself. This act alone makes your mind more focused on the way forward.

How do you get more protein?

The best sources of protein are meats, fish, eggs and dairy products. They have all the essential amino acids that your body needs. You can also consider adding in vegetables, nuts, seeds and oats. Remember this is not a diet but a journey of change and understanding. There is no reason to get hung up on what you are eating and its calorific content and the like. Just be aware that by increasing certain foods and including them in to your daily food intake and on a regular basis, you will start to notice the difference. *Now you take a look at the other food groups like carbs and fats. Take an interest. It's your body and your life. Live it in a healthy body.*

Choose foods that will help to speed up your metabolism like cinnamon, ginger, oats, mango, papaya, green tea, water, high citrus fruits, salmon, tuna, onion, garlic, broccoli, beetroot, salad stuff like rocket leaves.

Leave out the foods that will slow you down like wheat based products and alcohol. Do Tiny Noticeable Things to your diet over time. TNT your food and watch the inches and pounds begin to drop!

Chapter 10

Who We Are and What People Are Saying

"It's more than just a weight loss course, I feel better about everything. Last week was a stressful week at work and at home but I coped much better with it and did not use food as a stress buster at all ☺. "

"In the past I've only had enough will power to resist my urges for a few weeks but it has always been a battle. Now I go to the cookie aisle because of habit but my response is I don't actually want them! I want to go home and have dinner!"

"This has given me the tools to take back control and change my bad habits into good ones without feeling that I am depriving myself."

"I've stopped snacking by drinking water when I get the urge to snack."
"Outlook more positive, more energy and enthusiasm, feel happier."

"I'm a lot more active, drink 6-8 bottles of water a day, I don't drink coffee and only drink green tea. I also drink juice. I used to drink a lot of alcohol and now I don't drink any at all ☺. I feel so much better. Thank you!"

"I drink a lot more water than I ever have before, I have started leaving food on my plate which is unheard of for me."

"Hi, I just want to let you know I have now lost a total of 31.5 inches off of my body and lost almost 2 stone! I go on my holiday in just over a week's time and thanks to you I'm going to put a bikini on for the first time in years :) I feel so much better about myself and my heath is better too. I have recommended this programme to all of my friends, thank you so much, I'm never going to get out of shape again, you have given me the confidence to stick with this, it's so natural I don't feel like I'm doing anything ☺. Thank you!!!!!"

These are just a few extracts of the emails we get on a regular basis from real people just like you. People who have started to change the way they THINK, MOVE AND EAT on a regular basis.

You have read this book to here so understand this;

The same process has already begun to happen to you.

"Change the way you think, eat and move. Make small changes and watch the big results start to happen."

About The Authors

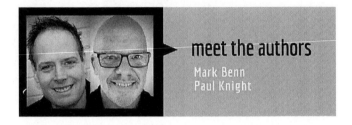

We coach people who struggle to lose weight, are totally over dieting and desperately need something different to happen with their lives.

Between us we have 50 years of experience and qualifications in health and fitness, behavioural change and weight loss. Using our expertise in NLP, hypnosis, food and fitness, we are fast becoming the go-to people for those who really want to look and feel their best.

Paul Knight

NLP Practitioner, Certified Fitness Trainer and Weight Loss Adviser

"I was a slip of lad, just 21, when I started my own journey into the world of health and fitness. All lycra-clad and hair, to the present day some 36 years later. During this time I have taught overseas, owned my own gym, and been at the forefront of community health to name a few things and enjoyed every minute of it. I am proud to have helped hundreds of people grow and develop their lives through being active.

I have to say here, I am frustrated with the way fitness has developed in recent years. I think I'm getting more anti-industry as I get older. It's a huge business these days and it's missing the point. You don't have to conform to it to be fit and healthy. That's why I love being involved with the people I deal with on a day to day basis now at Slimthinkers.

When I'm not sharing everything I know with those that need it, I'm watching my favourite rugby team – Leicester Tigers - or dancing at a Northern Soul 'do'. I once travelled around the world for 7 years. Oh, and I paint, art not decorating."

Mark Benn

Master level NLP and Hypnosis, Behavioural Change and Weight Loss Expert

"I am fascinated with what makes people tick, why we do what we do when we know what we are doing is going to create a negative outcome. The mind has always been an area which has excited me. From an early age I knew that I wanted to be involved in change work so I went down the line of corporate training, working as a consultant with some of the biggest companies in the UK, but this wasn't me. I liked seeing real people make real changes in their private lives, nothing beats the feeling when you see a person change their way of thinking before your eyes. So I have been running a busy clinic for many years with clients coming to see me from all walks of life and from all over the country.

When I'm not with clients or working with Paul, I'm usually looking after the kids and animals, twin girls, a 3 legged cat and chickens. I love life, enjoy playing the guitar and best of all family time."

Additional Resources

There are many ways in which we can help you move forward in your life, fitness and your weight loss goals. These include private one to one coaching, online courses delivered via video and audio and our downloadable hypnosis support. We look forward to hearing from you and helping you on your journey.

For more information please visit
www.slimthinkers.com

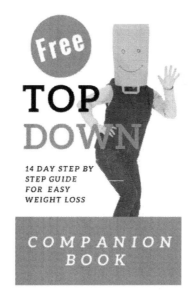

Don't forget to get your free copy of your companion book!

***www.slimthinkers.com/top-companion-course-book*)**

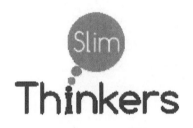

© <u>slimthinkers Ltd</u>

Printed in Great Britain
by Amazon